NAVIGATING ANGIOSARCOMA WITH CONFIDENCE AND CARE

Empowering Strategies For Confronting Cancer Head-On With Ease And Support For Healing And Holistic Wellness

DR. WESLEY IAN

DISCLAIMER

The information in this book is not meant to replace professional medical advice, diagnosis, or treatment; rather, it is meant mainly for general informational reasons. If you have any questions about a medical problem, you should always consult your doctor or another trained health expert. Don't ever discount expert medical advice or put off getting it because of something you've read in this book.

Any negative effects or repercussions arising from the usage of the material provided herein are not the responsibility of the book's author or publisher. It should be noted by readers that the material in this book is not all-inclusive and might not address every facet of the subject. Furthermore, new research may have an impact on how health concerns are understood or treated because medical knowledge is always changing.

No particular test, treatment, method, or product mentioned in this book is endorsed or promoted by the author or publisher. The reader assumes all risk associated with using the information included in this book.

Before making any big decisions regarding your health, it's crucial to speak with a licensed healthcare provider. The relationship between a patient and their healthcare practitioner should not be replaced by this book, nor is it meant to offer medical advice.

The opinions presented in this book are the author's and may not necessarily represent those of the publisher. Any errors, omissions, or inaccuracies in the information in this book are not the responsibility of the author or publisher.

It is recommended that readers independently confirm any information contained in this book and speak with a healthcare provider about their specific medical needs and state of health.

TABLE OF CONTENTS

CHAPTER ONE 12

THE INTRODUCTION TO ANGIOSARCOMA.............................12

KNOWLEDGE OF ANGIOSARCOMA 12

THE VALUE OF HANDLING ANGIOSARCOMA WITH CARE AND.........13

CHAPTER TWO 16

DESCRIBE ANGIOSARCOMA. 16

TYPES AND DEFINITIONS OF ANGIOSARCOMA 16

THE RATE AND FREQUENCY 17

REASONS AND DANGER ELEMENTS 17

SIGNS AND TIMELY IDENTIFICATION..................................18

CHAPTER THREE 20

IDENTIFYING ANGIOSARCOMA. 20

IMAGING AND MEDICAL TESTS 20

PROCEDURES FOR BIOPSIES 21

ANALYZING THE DIAGNOSIS OUTCOMES.............................21

LOOKING FOR SECOND OPINIONS 22

CHAPTER FOUR 24

OPTIONS FOR TREATMENT 24

OPERATION 24

RADIATION TREATMENT 24

CHEMOTHERAPY 25

PERSONALIZED TREATMENT 25

IMMUNOTHERAPY 26

CLINICAL INVESTIGATIONS 26

COMPLEMENTARY AND INTEGRATIVE THERAPIES 27

CHAPTER FIVE...28

MAKING TREATMENT DECISIONS 28

PUTTING TOGETHER A MEDICAL TEAM 28

COMPREHENDING TREATMENT PROGRAMS 29

KEEPING BENEFITS AND RISKS IN CHECK 29

SUPPORT FOR MAKING DECISIONS..30

CHAPTER SIX..32

CONTROLLING ADVERSE REACTIONS...32

COMMON SIDE EFFECTS OF TREATMENT FOR ANGIOSARCOMA 32

TECHNIQUES FOR HANDLING ADVERSE EFFECTS............................33

INTERACTION WITH MEDICAL PROFESSIONALS................................34

CHAPTER SEVEN 36

MENTAL AND EMOTIONAL ASSISTANCE 36

MANAGING A DIAGNOSIS: 36

PUTTING TOGETHER A SUPPORT NETWORK....................................37

WELL-BEING AND MENTAL HEALTH..37

HANDLING DEPRESSION AND ANXIETY 38

CHAPTER EIGHT 40

NUTRITION AND LIFESTYLE 40

THE VALUE OF LEADING A HEALTHFUL LIFESTYLE 40

PHYSICAL ACTIVITY AND EXERCISE..40

DIETARY AND NUTRITIONAL CONSIDERATIONS...............................41

INCLUDING WELLNESS TECHNIQUES 42

CHAPTER NINE 44

RESILIENCE AND CONTINUED CARE 44

    LIFE AFTER TREATMENT 44

    SURVIVORSHIP PLANS 45

    LONG-TERM FOLLOW-UP 46

CHAPTER TEN 48

  RESOURCES AND ADVOCACY 48

    TAKING UP YOUR DEFENSE 48

    GETTING IN TOUCH WITH SUPPORT SERVICES 49

    ESTABLISHING CONTACT WITH PATIENT ADVOCACY GROUPS 49

    ONLINE FORUMS AND COMMUNITIES 50

ABOUT THE BOOK

An excellent resource that covers the intricacies of angiosarcoma in detail is Navigating Angiosarcoma with Confidence and Care. The book begins by setting the scene by explaining its goal and stressing how important it is to comprehend and treat angiosarcoma with caution and confidence. The writers stress the value of this manual as a source of information and assistance for people traveling the difficult path of angiosarcoma.

To answer the central issue, "What is Angiosarcoma?" It examines the disease's several forms, incidence, prevalence, etiology, and risk factors. These fundamental insights provide a solid grasp of the illness and form the basis for the ensuing chapters. Patients and medical professionals can benefit from the emphasis on symptoms and early detection.

Subsequently, this book walks readers through the process of diagnosis by explaining biopsy techniques, medical testing, and how to interpret test results. To promote an informed and proactive approach to diagnosis—a critical step in the management of angiosarcomas—the chapter strongly pushes for getting second opinions.

Treatment choices and the process of making treatment selections are covered in this book. The book offers a thorough review of everything from immunotherapy to surgery, enabling readers to make knowledgeable decisions about their care. It also emphasizes how crucial it is to assemble a medical team, comprehend treatment regimens, and weigh the advantages and disadvantages of each option.

The practical aspects of caring for angiosarcoma patients are covered in the following chapters. In this book, side effect management is covered. Coping mechanisms are offered, and the importance of having good contact with healthcare practitioners is emphasized. An in-depth discussion of emotional and psychological support is covered in this book, which also acknowledges the effect of diagnosis on mental health and provides advice on creating a strong support network.

With an emphasis on the significance of healthy living, exercise, and nutrition in the setting of angiosarcoma, this book turns the attention to lifestyle and nutrition. The book incorporates wellness practices into the debate, so acknowledging the holistic nature of care.

This book delves into survivorship and follow-up care, providing insight into what happens after treatment, recurrence monitoring, and creating strategies for survivorship. In conclusion, this book explores advocacy and resources, enabling people to take on the role of their advocates, obtain assistance, and establish connections with online communities and patient advocacy groups.

Navigating Angiosarcoma with Confidence and Care is essentially an all-inclusive manual that goes beyond the disease's clinical features. It gives people the information, resources, and psychological support they need to face the complex terrain of angiosarcoma with fortitude and assurance.

CHAPTER ONE

THE INTRODUCTION TO ANGIOSARCOMA

KNOWLEDGE OF ANGIOSARCOMA

Angiosarcoma is an uncommon and highly aggressive kind of cancer that develops from the cells lining lymphatic or blood arteries. This cancer can develop in the skin, soft tissues, breast, or internal organs, among other sections of the body. Investigating the intricacies of angiosarcoma's pathophysiology, diagnosis, and treatment is necessary to comprehend the condition. Understanding the complexities of angiosarcoma becomes essential for medical professionals, patients, and their families due to its uncommon nature and range of symptoms.

The rare cancer's tendency for fast growth and potential for metastasis provides special problems. Angiosarcoma differs from other forms of sarcomas in that its pathophysiology is typified by aberrant and growing lymphatic or blood vessel cells.

To create more specialized and efficient treatment plans, scientists and medical professionals are always trying to understand the molecular and genetic components of angiosarcoma.

THE VALUE OF HANDLING ANGIOSARCOMA WITH CARE AND CONFIDENCE

It is crucial to navigate angiosarcoma with confidence and care; this cannot be emphasized enough. Healthcare professionals must handle the diagnosis and treatment of angiosarcoma with compassion and skill due to its rarity. Because this cancer is so uncommon, it emphasizes how crucial it is for researchers, patient advocacy organizations, and medical professionals to work together to increase knowledge and enhance patient outcomes.

Navigating the path of angiosarcoma can be physically and emotionally challenging for individuals and their families. Because Angiosarcoma is a rare disease, people who have it may feel alone, and alone, thus they need to find a support system.

As they help patients navigate the complex world of treatment options, possible side effects, and the overall impact on quality of life, patients must have complete confidence in the medical team and care providers.

Furthermore, research and innovation are areas where confidence is crucial for managing angiosarcoma. It is imperative to pursue the ongoing investigation of innovative treatments, customized medicine methodologies, and supportive care tactics to improve the prognosis and standard of living for those impacted by this difficult illness.

Trust in clinical trials and research projects can lead to discoveries that could result in better therapies and higher survival rates.

Our knowledge of angiosarcoma is still developing and necessitates a thorough approach from researchers, medical experts, and those who are impacted. It is important to acknowledge the emotional and social parts of the trip in addition to the medical ones to navigate Angiosarcoma with confidence and care.

It is imperative that medical professionals, researchers, and the community at large work together to advance understanding, improve treatment approaches, and eventually improve outcomes for patients with this uncommon and aggressive malignancy.

CHAPTER TWO

DESCRIBE ANGIOSARCOMA

TYPES AND DEFINITIONS OF ANGIOSARCOMA

Angiosarcoma is an uncommon and highly aggressive kind of cancer that starts in the lymphatic or blood vessels' inner lining. It belongs to the class of malignancies known as soft tissue sarcomas, which arise in the body's soft tissues, including blood vessels, muscles, and tendons. The word "angio" describes blood arteries, emphasizing where this malignancy is primarily found. Angiosarcomas can develop in the skin, liver, breast, and deep soft tissues, among other regions of the body.

Angiosarcoma comes in various forms, each of which affects different bodily parts. Skin cancer known as cutaneous angiosarcoma typically affects the head and neck. Breast angiosarcoma occurs in the breast tissue, whereas soft tissue angiosarcoma affects the deep soft tissues. Hepatic angiosarcoma is another kind that develops in the liver. Despite having a vascular basis in common, these subtypes have different clinical characteristics and can need different treatment modalities.

THE RATE AND FREQUENCY

Compared to more prevalent tumors, angiosarcoma has a comparatively low incidence and frequency. It is difficult to compile extensive statistics on its occurrence because of its rarity. The precise subtype and the tumor's anatomical location affect the occurrence. For example, hepatic angiosarcoma is less prevalent and typically affects younger people, but cutaneous angiosarcoma is more commonly identified in older people, usually in their 60s or 70s. Although rare, angiosarcoma can be extremely aggressive and difficult to cure, which adds to the disease's profound effects on those who are afflicted.

REASONS AND DANGER ELEMENTS

Research on angiosarcoma is hampered by the condition's rarity and incomplete understanding of its etiology. Nonetheless, several risk factors have been found. There has been evidence linking the development of vinyl chloride and thorium dioxide exposure to a higher incidence of angiosarcoma. Furthermore, there is a proven risk factor for the formation of angiosarcoma in the irradiated area—prior radiation therapy, especially for other tumors. Given that certain gene mutations have been connected to angiosarcoma cases, genetic factors may be involved.

SIGNS AND TIMELY IDENTIFICATION

Angiosarcoma symptoms might change based on where the tumor is located. Patients may notice the appearance of bruise-like lesions on their skin, usually on the face or scalp, when they have cutaneous angiosarcoma. Soft tissue angiosarcoma may appear as a bulge or deep-seated tumor. Skin changes or a lump in the breast are two possible symptoms of breast angiosarcoma. Although uncommon, hepatic angiosarcoma can result in swelling, pain in the abdomen, and other liver-related symptoms.

For optimal results and angiosarcoma treatment to be successful, early discovery is essential. However, the lack of specificity in the symptoms and the unusual character of the ailment can cause a delay in diagnosis. Imaging tests, such as CT or MRI scans, and biopsies to confirm the existence of angiosarcoma are examples of diagnostic techniques. A thorough assessment and suitable management of angiosarcoma necessitate immediate medical attention and consultation with professionals due to its aggressive nature.

CHAPTER THREE

IDENTIFYING ANGIOSARCOMA
IMAGING AND MEDICAL TESTS

An extensive diagnostic process involving numerous medical tests and imaging examinations is required to diagnose angiosarcoma. The presence of angiosarcoma, a rare and aggressive type of cancer that starts in the blood vessels, must be determined with the use of these instruments. To guarantee precise and trustworthy results, medical experts usually use a variety of diagnostic techniques.

Imaging and medical testing are essential in the early diagnosis of angiosarcoma. Imaging tests including computed tomography (CT) scans, magnetic resonance imaging (MRI), and angiography aid in the visualization of the damaged areas and offer important details regarding the size of the tumor.

These non-invasive methods help identify the tumor, measure its size, and evaluate how it affects the surrounding tissues.

PROCEDURES FOR BIOPSIES

The foundation of diagnosing angiosarcoma is biopsy techniques. During a biopsy, a pathologist removes a tiny sample of tissue from the suspected tumor and examines it under a microscope. Tissue samples can be obtained by standard techniques such as core needle biopsy and surgical biopsy.

The location and accessibility of the tumor are among the criteria that influence the biopsy procedure choice. A conclusive diagnosis of angiosarcoma can be made by the histological evaluation of the biopsy sample, which evaluates the unique properties of the cancer cells.

ANALYZING THE DIAGNOSIS OUTCOMES

It takes the knowledge of a multidisciplinary team of medical specialists to interpret diagnosis results. To confirm the presence of angiosarcoma, pathologists examine the cellular morphology and features in the biopsy samples. Radiologists use imaging study interpretation to determine the location of tumors and how they affect nearby structures.

This combined data is used by oncologists to identify the cancer's stage, which informs prognosis and therapy choices.

LOOKING FOR SECOND OPINIONS

Getting second opinions is a wise step in the angiosarcoma diagnosis procedure. Because this cancer is so uncommon and complicated, getting a second opinion from a sarcoma expert or specialized oncologist can offer valuable information and guarantee the most correct diagnosis.

In addition to providing patients with a more thorough grasp of their disease, second views may serve to validate the first diagnosis and present alternate viewpoints of available treatments.

A variety of medical tests, imaging examinations, biopsy techniques, and professional interpretation of the results are used in the diagnosis of angiosarcoma. For angiosarcoma to be correctly diagnosed and staged, pathologists, radiologists, and oncologists must work together.

CHAPTER FOUR
OPTIONS FOR TREATMENT
OPERATION

Surgery is an essential part of medical therapy for many diseases, including cancer. To stop or slow the disease's spread, tumors or other abnormal tissues must be removed from the body. Depending on the kind and stage of cancer, different surgical techniques are used; technological developments have produced less intrusive methods that speed up recovery and lessen the toll taken on the patient's general health.

RADIATION TREATMENT

High doses of ionizing radiation are used in radiation treatment to specifically target and kill cancer cells. This therapy can be used internally by putting radioactive materials right at the tumor location, or externally by utilizing devices outside the body. The intention is to harm cancer cells' DNA so that it can't divide and proliferate. Depending on the particulars of the malignancy, radiation therapy is frequently employed as a stand-alone treatment or in combination with surgery.

CHEMOTHERAPY

Drugs are used in chemotherapy to either kill or stop the spread of cancer cells throughout the body. Chemotherapy is a systemic treatment that can reach cancer cells anywhere in the body, unlike radiation therapy or surgery. When metastasis is likely or has already occurred, it is frequently used. Chemotherapy is an effective treatment, but it can also have negative effects on healthy, normal cells that divide quickly, such as those in the bone marrow and digestive system.

PERSONALIZED TREATMENT

Targeted therapy targets particular chemicals that are essential to the development and spread of cancer cells. As opposed to chemotherapy, which damages both diseased and healthy cells, targeted therapy aims to specifically obstruct the mechanisms that support the growth and survival of cancer cells. This strategy seeks to limit adverse consequences while minimizing damage to good tissues. The efficacy of targeted therapy is contingent upon the particular molecular features of the malignancy and is frequently utilized in combination with other treatments.

IMMUNOTHERAPY

Through immunotherapy, cancer cells are identified and eradicated by the body's immune system. This therapy strengthens the immune response or breaks down the defenses cancer cells put up to keep the immune system from recognizing them. Immunotherapy can produce long-term remission and has demonstrated impressive success in treating several cancer types. Adoptive cell treatment, cancer vaccines, and immune checkpoint inhibitors are a few examples of different forms of immunotherapy.

CLINICAL INVESTIGATIONS

To increase the possibilities for treating cancer, clinical trials are crucial. These patient-participated studies assess the efficacy and safety of novel treatments or combinations of treatments. Clinical trials offer insightful information about novel strategies that might eventually become accepted as standard therapy. To receive state-of-the-art care and further medical research, patients might think about taking part in clinical trials.

COMPLEMENTARY AND INTEGRATIVE THERAPIES

Complementary and integrative therapies cover a broad spectrum of methods that extend beyond traditional medical care. Dietary adjustments, acupuncture, massage, yoga, and meditation are a few examples of these. These therapies can help manage symptoms, promoting overall well-being, and improving quality of life, even though they are not commonly utilized as main cancer treatments. The purpose of integrating complementary and integrative therapies with conventional medical treatments is to address the psychological, spiritual, and emotional elements of cancer therapy.

CHAPTER FIVE
MAKING TREATMENT DECISIONS
PUTTING TOGETHER A MEDICAL TEAM

Making decisions on a patient's course of treatment requires putting together a comprehensive healthcare team that works together to handle a patient's condition in its entirety. Specialists, general practitioners, nurses, and other medical personnel usually make up this team. Every member adds a different area of expertise, which helps to create a comprehensive plan for patient care. When assembling a healthcare team, it is important to take into account the patient's medical background, present state of health, and unique obstacles associated with their illness.

Team members must effectively coordinate and communicate with one another to guarantee that the patient receives comprehensive care that is tailored to meet their specific needs.

COMPREHENDING TREATMENT PROGRAMS

Learning all there is to know about the suggested treatment plans is essential to making informed treatment decisions. Healthcare providers create customized strategies called treatment plans to address the health conditions of their patients. A variety of interventions are covered by these programs, including prescription drugs, surgeries, lifestyle adjustments, and therapeutic interventions. It is important for patients and their caregivers to actively communicate with their healthcare team to understand the reasoning behind each treatment plan component. This comprehension facilitates well-informed decision-making, enabling patients to take an active role in their care and follow the recommended course of action.

KEEPING BENEFITS AND RISKS IN CHECK

Making treatment decisions requires a careful balancing act between possible dangers and benefits. Healthcare professionals need to carefully consider the potential advantages of a given treatment choice against any related hazards. The patient's medical history, current state of health, and personal preferences are all taken into account. In turn, patients must be made aware of the potential drawbacks, difficulties, and anticipated results of various therapy alternatives. Open communication between patients and healthcare providers is necessary to balance risks and benefits and facilitate shared decision-making that is in line with the patient's objectives and values.

SUPPORT FOR MAKING DECISIONS

Making treatment selections can be difficult, particularly when there are a lot of options and complicated medical facts to consider. To help patients and their families make decisions that are consistent with their beliefs and preferences, decision-making support is essential. This support can take many different forms, including shared decision-making conversations with healthcare providers, counseling, and decision aids. When making decisions together, patients and healthcare providers take into account each other's individual needs, preferences, and goals. This process is known as shared decision-making. Giving patients the knowledge and resources they require improves their capacity to actively engage in the decision-making process and increases their sense of assurance throughout the treatment they have selected.

Making judgments about treatment entails assembling a strong healthcare team, comprehending treatment strategies, weighing the advantages and disadvantages, and getting assistance with decision-making. Through active patient participation in their care, this multimodal approach guarantees more individualized and successful treatment outcomes.

CHAPTER SIX

CONTROLLING ADVERSE REACTIONS

COMMON SIDE EFFECTS OF TREATMENT FOR ANGIOSARCOMA

Treatment for angiosarcoma patients may cause a variety of typical side effects, which might differ in severity and length. Fatigue is a common side effect that can negatively affect everyday activities and quality of life. Excessive fatigue is frequently a result of the demanding nature of cancer therapies like radiation and chemotherapy. Other common adverse effects include nausea and vomiting, especially after chemotherapy sessions. Antiemetic drugs might be recommended to address these symptoms and enhance the therapeutic process in general.

Hair loss is another frequent adverse effect of angiosarcoma treatment, and it can be emotionally taxing for patients. People may find it easier to adjust to the changes in their looks if they realize that this is a transitory part of the treatment process. Furthermore, patients may notice changes in their appetite and weight as a result of therapy side effects or the emotional toll that receiving a diagnosis might have. During this time, it can be helpful to keep a balanced diet and ask healthcare professionals for nutritional advice.

TECHNIQUES FOR HANDLING ADVERSE EFFECTS

A diversified strategy that takes into account the patient's emotional and physical health is necessary to manage the negative effects of angiosarcoma treatment. People need the support of friends and family to get through the difficult times that come with receiving therapy. Building a solid support network can offer consolation on an emotional level as well as useful support when one is more vulnerable. Open conversation about wants and feelings is a healthy way to build understanding and a sense of connection with those closest to you.

Complementary therapies can assist in managing stress and enhance general well-being. Examples of these therapies include yoga, meditation, and acupuncture. These methods might help promote a more optimistic outlook in addition to relieving bodily discomfort. It is recommended that patients investigate different coping techniques to determine which ones most closely align with their personal preferences and requirements.

Effectively identifying and treating side effects also depends on keeping lines of communication open with healthcare practitioners. Medical practitioners can modify treatment plans in response to the patient's tolerance and response, as well as provide insightful information about supportive care measures that are now available. It is imperative for patients to rapidly report any new or worsening symptoms, as prompt action can frequently stop side effects from getting worse and enhance the patient experience overall.

INTERACTION WITH MEDICAL PROFESSIONALS

While treating angiosarcoma, good communication between patients and medical professionals is essential to delivering the best possible care and controlling side effects. Patients can voice concerns, ask questions, and actively engage in therapeutic decision-making when trustworthy and transparent communication is established. Patients can discuss symptoms, treatment progress, and any emergent side effects during regularly scheduled sessions.

Patients should keep a thorough log of all the symptoms they have, including the beginning, length, and severity, to give medical professionals a thorough picture of their overall health. When necessary, this information allows for more precise assessments and treatment plan modifications. Since the psychosocial components of cancer treatment are critical to general health, it is imperative that patients be open and honest about their emotional state.

In turn, healthcare personnel are essential in promoting good communication between patients and themselves by making sure patients are aware of their treatment options, possible side effects, and available resources for support. By allowing patients to actively engage in their care, collaborative decision-making improves patient outcomes and the overall treatment experience.

CHAPTER SEVEN

MENTAL AND EMOTIONAL ASSISTANCE

MANAGING A DIAGNOSIS:

Getting a diagnosis can be a very difficult emotional experience, especially if it concerns one's physical or mental health. Navigating a spectrum of emotions, from shock and denial to acceptance and adaptability, is part of coping with a diagnosis. It is critical to understand that everyone's coping mechanism is different and that there is no one-size-fits-all solution.

During this time, emotional support from friends, family, or mental health specialists can be quite beneficial. Comprehending the diagnosis, compiling data, and requesting clarification from medical professionals are crucial phases in the coping mechanism. A more resilient coping strategy can also be facilitated by taking proactive measures and emphasizing self-care.

PUTTING TOGETHER A SUPPORT NETWORK

Developing a strong support network is essential for mental and emotional health. Family, friends, coworkers, and mental health experts who provide comprehension, empathy, and encouragement can all be considered members of a support system. Opening channels of communication within the support system makes people feel heard and validated and helps them feel connected. Beyond only providing emotional support, practical aid like assistance with daily activities or transportation can lessen some of the responsibilities brought on by difficult situations. Understanding the value of mutually beneficial connections, in which people support one another's well-being, fortifies the support network as a whole and increases resiliency in the face of adversity.

WELL-BEING AND MENTAL HEALTH

Sustaining mental health and general well-being necessitates a multifaceted, comprehensive approach.

This is taking good care of one's physical health by engaging in regular exercise, eating a balanced diet, and getting enough sleep. Including mindfulness exercises, like yoga or meditation, can help people become more emotionally resilient and reduce stress. Creating a happy and supportive social network and engaging in joyful and fulfilling activities are important for mental health. Getting professional assistance, such as therapy or counseling, can give you useful tools for understanding emotions, controlling stress, and promoting personal development. It's critical to understand that maintaining mental health is a continuous process that calls for constant attention and support.

HANDLING DEPRESSION AND ANXIETY

Common psychological disorders like anxiety and depression can have a serious negative effect on a person's quality of life. A multifaceted strategy is needed to address these problems, which may include social support, lifestyle changes, and therapeutic therapies. The thought patterns and behaviors linked to anxiety and depression can be effectively understood and managed by patients with the aid of evidence-based therapies such as cognitive-behavioral therapy (CBT). Modifications in lifestyle, such as consistent exercise, enough sleep, and a balanced diet, can improve mood and reduce symptoms. An important defense against the isolating consequences of these situations is social support from friends, family, and professional networks. For certain people, medication that is prescribed and overseen by medical professionals may be an important part of their treatment. Crucially, lowering stigma and encouraging candid discussions about mental health help create a society that is more understanding and supportive of people who are struggling with anxiety and despair.

CHAPTER EIGHT

NUTRITION AND LIFESTYLE

THE VALUE OF LEADING A HEALTHFUL LIFESTYLE

It is impossible to overestimate the significance of leading a healthy lifestyle because it affects all facets of one's well-being, including mental, emotional, and physical health. Living a healthy lifestyle is making deliberate decisions that support general vitality and longevity, not just the absence of disease. A healthy lifestyle is essential for reducing the risk of chronic illnesses, building resilience, and enhancing life quality. It includes a well-balanced mix of mindful wellness activities, a healthy diet, and frequent physical activity.

PHYSICAL ACTIVITY AND EXERCISE

Physical activity and exercise are essential for encouraging a healthy lifestyle. Frequent exercise enhances cardiovascular health, fortifies muscles and bones, and elevates mental well-being in addition to helping one maintain a healthy weight. Physical activity lowers stress and anxiety by releasing endorphins, the body's natural mood enhancers. To get the most out of an active lifestyle, discover fun methods to keep active, whether it's through weight training, yoga, tai chi, or cardiovascular exercises like jogging or cycling.

DIETARY AND NUTRITIONAL CONSIDERATIONS

Dietary guidelines and nutrition are essential components of a healthy lifestyle. The body gets the vital nutrients, vitamins, and minerals it needs from a well-balanced diet to perform at its best. A healthy diet emphasizes whole foods including fruits, vegetables, whole grains, and lean meats, and minimizes processed and sugary meals. Water is necessary for healthy digestion, vitamin absorption, and the body's removal of toxins, so staying properly hydrated is just as vital. In addition to having an impact on physical health, nutrition is also very important for mental and emotional wellness.

INCLUDING WELLNESS TECHNIQUES

Complementing the physical aspects of healthy living is the incorporation of wellness activities into daily life. Mental and emotional balance is enhanced by practices like mindfulness, meditation, and stress-reduction strategies. Getting enough sleep is essential for overall health because it gives the body time to relax, heal, and regenerate. A holistic approach to well-being includes controlling stress, cultivating connections, and fostering a supportive social environment. Combining these strategies increases life happiness overall, builds resilience, and lowers the likelihood of burnout.

Let's sum up by saying that healthy living is a broad notion that includes thoughtful wellness habits, a balanced diet, and physical activity. Setting these things in order of importance leads to a robust and active lifestyle that enhances longevity and improves quality of life. Committing to living a healthy lifestyle can pay off in the long run by improving one's physical and mental health.

CHAPTER NINE

RESILIENCE AND CONTINUED CARE

LIFE AFTER TREATMENT

Transitioning to a new normal following cancer treatment is a crucial stage in a survivor's journey, characterized by feelings of relief as well as difficulty. When treatment is over, a range of feelings is frequently experienced, including happiness, thankfulness, and even worry about the future.

Survivorship emphasizes the significance of overall health by encompassing the time after active treatment. People may have changes in their physical, mental, and social status, necessitating continued assistance in overcoming obstacles that arise after therapy.

A vital component of survivability is vigilant surveillance for the recurrence of cancer. There is a chance of recurrence even with effective therapy, therefore routine check-ups and screenings are necessary. A mix of physical examinations, diagnostic testing, and reviews of medical history are used by healthcare providers to identify any recurrence signals early on when they can be more effectively managed. Patients are frequently informed about possible symptoms and urged to report any strange changes as soon as they occur. In addition to looking for potential recurrences, the monitoring method tries to handle new health concerns and provide all-encompassing treatment catered to the specific requirements of the survivor.

SURVIVORSHIP PLANS

During the post-treatment period, survivorship plans are essential because they give people a road map for managing their health and well-being. These individualized plans usually contain information regarding the cancer diagnosis, the course of therapy, and suggestions for aftercare. Survivorship plans are joint initiatives by survivors, their support systems, and medical professionals. They include ways to manage possible long-term adverse effects, keep up a healthy lifestyle, and take care of emotional and mental well-being.

Through the promotion of transparent communication and collaborative decision-making, survivorship plans enable individuals to take an active role in their continued care.

LONG-TERM FOLLOW-UP

After cancer treatment is over, people's requirements change and long-term follow-up care is a crucial part of survival. It focuses on observing and meeting these needs. This extended phase acknowledges that the effects of cancer persist long after treatment has concluded. Regular health examinations, screenings, and consultations are part of long-term follow-up, which aims to identify and treat any emerging health issues as well as detect and manage treatment side effects.

During this stage, the importance of health promotion and illness-preventive techniques increases, highlighting a proactive approach to preserving general well-being.

Adjusting to a new normal following cancer treatment is a dynamic process. Survivorship, recurrence monitoring, survivorship strategies, and long-term follow-up care all play a part in providing a thorough and patient-centered approach. Every person's journey through survivorship is different, which emphasizes the value of continued assistance and cooperation between survivors, medical professionals, and the larger support system.

CHAPTER TEN

RESOURCES AND ADVOCACY

TAKING UP YOUR DEFENSE

In the field of healthcare, taking charge of your advocacy is a crucial and empowering idea. It entails actively contributing to your health and well-being, being aware of your medical situation, and taking part in the decision-making processes surrounding it. People must educate themselves on their medical history, available treatments, and possible outcomes to be successful self-advocates.

This can entail getting a second opinion, raising concerns or preferences about treatment plans, and asking questions at doctor's appointments. People may make sure their voice is heard and have more effective and individualized healthcare experiences by adopting this proactive approach.

GETTING IN TOUCH WITH SUPPORT SERVICES

Making use of support services is essential when navigating intricate healthcare systems. A vast array of resources are included in support services, many of which are intended to help people deal with their health issues. Depending on the severity of the health problem, this can entail obtaining counseling, therapy, or rehabilitation treatments. In addition, government agencies, community organizations, and healthcare facilities may offer financial, practical, or emotional help. Acknowledging and availing of these services can considerably mitigate the stresses linked to health-related obstacles and enhance the general standard of living for people and their families.

ESTABLISHING CONTACT WITH PATIENT ADVOCACY GROUPS

Patient advocacy organizations are essential in promoting the welfare and rights of people dealing with certain medical conditions. For patients and their families, these organizations frequently offer a multitude of resources, information, and support systems. Making connections with these groups can provide a feeling of belonging, common ground, and insightful advice on how to manage a specific medical issue. Individuals can also obtain educational resources, take part in awareness campaigns, and support research projects targeted at improving therapies and discovering cures through advocacy groups. These organizations' collaborative style creates a supportive environment that enables people to overcome health difficulties more skillfully.

ONLINE FORUMS AND COMMUNITIES

Online forums and groups have become essential tools in the digital age for bringing people together who have similar health issues. These online forums give users a place to talk about their experiences, and trade knowledge, and offer emotional support. For people dealing with uncommon or persistent illnesses, online forums can be quite helpful as they foster a sense of community and lessen feelings of loneliness. But it's crucial to approach internet material with caution and confirm details with medical experts. Through engagement in these online groups, people can acquire knowledge about coping mechanisms, available treatments, and recent advancements in the industry. This, in turn, promotes a feeling of solidarity and self-determination among those facing comparable health experiences.